BreathWORK

Copyright © 2018 Gene Smithson

All rights reserved. No part of this publication may be reproduced, distributed or transmitted in any form or by any means, including photocopying, recording, or other electronic or mechanical methods, without the prior written permission of the publisher, except in the case of brief quotations embodied in critical reviews and certain other noncommercial uses permitted by copyright law. For permission requests, write to the publisher, addressed "Attention: Permissions Coordinator," at the address below:

Gene Smithson

803 Lambeth Lane

Austin Texas 78748

waldosmithson@yahoo.com

Cover and interior design by Gene Smithson

ISBN 9781798692349

First Edition

Disclaimer: Information in this book is distributed "As Is," without warranty. Nothing in this document constitutes a legal opinion nor should any of its contents be treated as such. Neither the authors nor the publisher shall have any liability with respect to information contained herein. Further, neither the author nor the publisher have any control over or assume any responsibility for websites or external resources referenced in this book. When it comes to martial arts, self-defense, violence, and related topics, no text, no matter how well written, can substitute for professional, hands-on instruction. The information contained in this manuscript is not to be taken as medical advice or a substitution for medical advice. Please consult with your Dr before beginning any exercise program. These materials should be used for academic study only

BreathWORK

Gene Smithson

Table of Contents

Introduction

The Two Minute Test

Belly Breathing

Beyond the Belly

Awareness Breathing

Stretching the Body (Pandiculation)

Standing BreathWORK

Empathy Breathing

Breathing Through the Mind

In One, Out One

Box Breathing

Triangle Breathing

Breath Holding as a Diagnostic

Pulse Point Breathing

Free Breathing

Conclusion

Introduction

When I was 14 years old, my first Karate teacher told me that breathing was the most important element of practice in martial arts. There were no follow up instructions, drills or exercises and it was never mentioned again.

As I "progressed" in my training journey, I came to believe that breathing was a catch all term for conditioning and cardiovascular workouts. Whenever someone became out of breath sparring or wrestling, it was clear that they needed more time running or on the bike to improve their "cardio".

As I continued my martial arts journey, I was simultaneously participating in triathlons, sometimes racing as many as 12 or 15 times a year. I completed several half Ironman races and the gorgeous Escape from Alcatraz triathlon which includes a lengthy swim in the chilly waters of San Francisco Bay. It was bewildering to me that I could perform these feats of endurance for hour upon hour yet, be out of breath within minutes whilst sparring or training martial arts. I was puzzled over how to increase my "cardio" because I was doing so much already and STILL I would "gas out" while grappling.

My first inkling that something different was called for was a roll with Carlos Machado. A roll is a light grappling or sparring session, it was definitely a light roll for Master Machado as he was still competing at a world class level and I was a newcomer in the world of Brazilian jiu jitsu. As we rolled, I could hear him almost whistling, this was done in strange rhythms and bursts and was clearly not song. I watched and listened as he worked through 15 people TWICE, match after match with seemingly no effort. I saw that while student after student gassed out or became exhausted, Carlos looked relaxed and was never out of breath. When asked about his whistling noises, he responded nonchalantly that he was breathing properly. It was clear to me that I was severely lacking in any understanding of breathing.

As my misconceptions and misunderstandings regarding breathing were being challenged on a deep level, I stumbled into an incredible encounter with a man who was to completely turn my ideas about breathing on their head. My personal exploration of martial art and breathing was about to take a much-needed turn.

Professor Teng Ying Bo is a qigong master from China.

In October of 2002 I traveled with a small group of Americans to Beijing, China. I had been training MMA and grappling and sparring regularly, even competing on several occasions. My shoulders were trashed, one was so damaged that I could barely lift my arm overhead. A good friend of mine was passing through Austin, Texas. Jesse had been living and training in China and Japan for many years and he was in the USA teaching a couple of seminars on qigong and Taoist yoga practices. When I talked to him about my shoulder he gave me a simple exercise to do and told me to do it 20 minutes a day. I call the exercise the teacup exercise as I am unsure of the actual name. At any rate, I performed the exercise mostly every day and a few times as many as 20 minutes, but I was pretty relaxed about the idea and skeptical that anything could help. I had already visited an orthopedic surgeon who recommended surgery and 12 months of rehab. Much to my surprise, within a couple of weeks my shoulder felt fine. Suddenly, I could do handstand presses whereas 2 weeks before I couldn't lift my arm over my head! The idea that a surgeon could be wrong and drastically so, really rocked my paradigm. It was this experience which left me open to traveling to China even though I myself had never studied any Chinese martial arts.

A few months after giving me the magic moves to heal my shoulder, Jesse contacted me again and suggested I accompany him and a group on a three-week trip to China to study at sacred Taoist sites and meet real qigong masters. I was highly skeptical, AND I was highly broke, seeing no way I could afford a trip to China on my nearly non-existent wages. As often happens in my life, fate intervened. Within a day of Jesse telling me about the trip to China a woman contacted me needing a quick paint job on a home she was selling. And, just like in the movies, the amount she offered was exactly what I needed to afford to go. To me it seemed like destiny, so I contacted Jesse, signed up for the trip and within a couple of weeks was on my way to China with a diverse group of folks I was soon to fall completely in love with. We shared many magical moments.

The first morning in Beijing I have described in SHOT: Healing Hurt, but to set the scene I was at Fragrant Hills Hotel in Beijing, China, a Frank Lloyd Wright-ish hotel set within the confines of a huge park. That first morning we were introduced to a qigong master...to this day I cannot remember his name, which is ironic because he really, really wanted to be remembered. The reason I cannot remember him is because a few minutes after his hour-long demonstration a teacher asked if we would like another lesson. We all quickly agreed that we would.

Professor Teng Ying Bo is a slight man, he may weigh 130 pounds, but I sort of doubt it. He showed up that morning in gold corduroy pants, a white turtleneck shirt and a pea coat. His hair was mussed from the 4-hour bus ride from his home to the park; the back had a cow lick which stood straight up in the air. I had at that time never met a man with such a quiet yet powerful presence. Some force field surrounded him, some energy emanated that elicited a refinement in all those who came near him. Years later I asked a friend who trained with Professor Teng if he had noticed anything unusual when he spent time with the professor...he laughed aloud because it was ALL so unusual, but he knew exactly what I meant. It was impossible to curse or even to have the feeling to curse in Prof. Teng's presence. Whatever he was putting out washed the perceptions and experiences of those around him to the point that those angry energies were just not possible. I saw it over and over when walking down the streets of Beijing. People would cease mid argument and look around in bewilderment as he passed, then moments later resume their loud, angry discourse. I called it his LOVE bubble and yes, I know how that sounds. If you can imagine it, I was a rather skeptical fellow, but what I saw and felt could not be denied by any truthful witness.

That first morning Professor Teng took our small group and walked us through the beginnings of a qigong practice. It was the opening day of a week of training that would radically alter my life, my training and my understanding of breath and its power. Some of the exercises he taught us will be described here in this book. No description can come close though, to illustrating the power, grace and kindness of the man I still consider my teacher. To truly know Professor Teng's genius you can travel to China and train with him yourself. He has a small clinic there and works with people just like you.

While in China I discovered several of the real deal, movie type masters that I had given up on. After over 20 years training in the USA I had never met anyone even close to the ideal master I was searching for, I had plenty of good teachers, but the masters as depicted in the Kung Fu series seemed to be non-existent. Professor Teng is the real deal and so are several other of the men I had the great good fortune to meet and train with while there. I'm not saying that level of skill doesn't exist here in the USA, I'm just saying that I personally never encountered a real master until I met Professor Teng Ying Bo. I am forever grateful for his commitment to breathwork and for introducing it to me in such a powerful way.

When I returned to America, I vowed to give up martial art…to be honest after what I experienced while in China, I thought that to continue my training here was just a waste of time. I stopped training martial art and devoted myself to finding a qigong teacher like Professor Teng. I could not find anyone like him anywhere and so several months later I wound up training Taijiquan with a beautiful human and amazing teacher by the name of Stan Rossi. Stan is gone now, but his kindness and compassion are ideals that I aspire to every day. Also, to my surprise, I discovered that taijiquan was a martial art and that I had not in fact given up martial art, only shifted temporarily to a different practice. Most people training taijiquan do not train it as a martial art, or if they do, they are not fighters and that is fine. For me, within a couple of months of beginning I realized, even more so than my teacher, that taijiquan is a real martial art. This was an interesting development for me in that it confirmed for me, that my personal path, was a martial one. I was back in the punch, kick, takedown and grapple world. This turned out to be most fortunate.

Vladimir Vasiliev is a master of martial art. When I saw him on the internet I immediately figured he was either the best I had ever seen, or he was a complete fraud. I had to find out which. These days it is common for people to watch a video clip on YouTube and determine that a martial artist is fake or, the real thing. It is easy to pronounce opinions and posit positions from a place of absolute ignorance or from a perspective that is so fundamentally different than the one being demonstrated that the observer is simply incapable of making a clear assessment. I urge anyone with doubts who is a sincere seeker to go find out for themselves. Vladimir is in Toronto, Canada, and he is the man who put it all together for me.

Breathing is moving is structural is relaxed, and doing it well makes you more competent at everything human.

Vladmir's work was the method I had searched for since the very beginning. Much of the work described in this book will be directly from him or extrapolated through my own practice and experience from exercises he has taught to me. After a lifetime of fog and smoke and mirrors, Vladimir Vasiliev put breath work into practice and into a method that will take anyone who tries it to levels they currently can only dream about.

The Two Minute Test

A few years back I had the privilege to train some of Austin, Texas' finest police officers. I had done a couple of large introductory seminars but now I was being offered the opportunity to teach every field training officer in Austin. The topic I chose was breathing. A fair number of my comrades and fellow instructors figured I was making a mistake. In the opinion of a lot of people, cops would never go for breathing exercises; too boring.

As it turned out the officers loved the material, were able to use it right away and rated the workshops very highly. So, how did I get the police to invest themselves in the training? I had one huge factor in my favor already, for these men and women violence was neither sport nor theoretical. They all had extensive experience in real world actual violence. This makes it easy for me. I can skip all the convincing and trying to educate about the reality of violent encounters and get right to work offering tools that work for those real situations.

And second, I use the two-minute test.

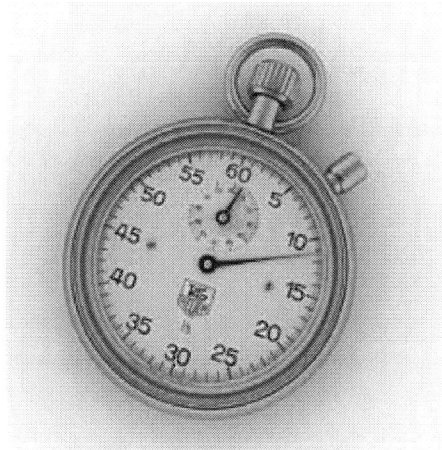

At the start of any breathwork seminar I have ever taught there is either severe skepticism or an idea that breathing exercises are some magical activity reserved for the almost enlightened. With the police, the officers were skeptical, these folks are forced to sit through seminars all the time that are taught by folks with no understanding of the jobs the police are tasked to do, and so predictably the officers were all glued to the walls of the room, no one venturing out in the open space where all manner of foolishness was likely to happen.

So, I just asked them to give me two minutes.

Try this exercise yourself or use it to introduce breathing practices to those who may be skeptical.

DRILL

Two minutes in the up position of a pushup or as we called it in the Navy, lean and rest. Some folks refer to it as a plank position. Ask the participants or yourself to record the level of difficulty. Some folks will make it the full two minutes, some will fall out early, doesn't matter, just ask them (or yourself) to give their best effort and record the level of difficulty.

When the two minutes is over; ask the participants to relax, lie down on their backs and recover for a bit. When ready to proceed, partner up if possible…if not you can use a bean bag or a book or any light weight object. Have your partners place one hand on your stomach and one on your chest. The purpose of the hands or the light objects is to provide a tactile target for your awareness. It is not to be heavy or restrictive.

Step 1

Breathe into the stomach but not the chest. The hand or the object placed on your stomach should rise on the inhale and fall on the exhale. The hand on the chest should remain motionless. Repeat for several breaths, a minimum of three will work.

If you have strong healthy people you can illustrate this principle by having a person lie on the other persons chest, restricting the movement there so that the only space available for breath is by relaxing the tummy and allowing space for the diaphragm muscle to move down into freely as the organs are massaged and gently moved aside on the inhale and then released to neutral on the exhale.

Step 2

Breathe and allow the chest to rise but not the tummy.

Sadly, this is how a lot of people breathe normally, using the intercostal and scalene muscles to breathe rather than the diaphragm. This has truly disastrous consequences as breathing this way tilts your physiology in favor of sympathetic nervous system (SNS) dominance rather than the parasympathetic nervous system (PSNS). In laymen's terms, this means you are breathing to keep yourself in the fight, flight or freeze state rather than the rest, digest and recover state.

Again, it is possible to use the partners body weight to restrict the ability to breathe by compromising the breather's ability to relax the stomach and use the diaphragm muscle.

Step 3

Breathe and create a wave. On the inhale the tummy rises first followed by the chest. On the exhale, the chest falls first, followed by the tummy thus creating a wave up and then down the front of the torso.

Some folks can do this right away, for some it takes a few tries to work out the coordination, be patient and explore.

Super advanced version of this part is a person stands on you with one foot on your tummy and one on your chest and you breathe into the space in between their feet. Please do not attempt this exercise without proper supervision, proper preparation and some really strong torso muscles.

Step 4

Turn face down on the floor and have partner place hands or light weight object on the kidney area. Breathe down low into the persons hands or your target objects. The viscera are pushed down when the diaphragm moves downward, if the muscles in the lower back are relaxed you can feel the kidney area swell with each inhale and release with each exhale. In many cases the person who has their hands there will feel a sensation similar to water moving through a hose, very interesting.

For this part of the exercise only very light breath targets should be used. Never press hard on anyone's lower back. The architecture of the lumbar region is not made to support weight from this direction.

Step 5

Place the hands on the upper back. Could be at shoulder blade level or higher, as if you were going to massage the persons trapezius muscles. Breath into the upper back and the trapezius area.

This upper back is very easy for most folks to access. The trapezius area is rather more advanced, and it is unlikely that untrained persons will be able to breathe here. With training it is no problem.

Once these exercises are completed I ask the person or you to consider this. You were definitely able to breathe into different areas of the body. Yes, air only goes into the lungs; however, by adjusting your focus and awareness you are able to move breath, not air, around to different body areas.

Now we need to see if breathing can give any tangible benefit.

DRILL

Please repeat the 2-minute plank hold. The instructions are, breathe fully as you hold the position. Breathe a little faster than normal, your body is working and needs the extra oxygen. As you feel tension arise in the various parts of your body use your new awareness and breathe into these areas. If your neck is tense, breathe into trapezius area. If your arms are feeling shaky, breathe into the chest or shoulder area; likewise, with lower back or stomach muscles.

To date, no one has not found the perceived effort to complete the plank to be much easier.

Ofttimes every person tasked would suddenly be able to maintain the plank for the entire 2 minutes. And I have been accused on many occasions of cheating the time on the second plank. I never have. It really does improve performance that much.

This is how I introduce breathwork. Right away I establish that it will be work, but that breathing can dramatically and immediately improve your actual physical performance. I let that idea sink in and then I ask as an aside how the person or people feel after breathing this way and performing the second plank position. Again, without exception, they report a more relaxed and calmer state. This is quite an important experience for law enforcement officers as they suffer tremendously from the effects of one of the most stressful jobs on the planet.

Belly Breathing (Softening the belly)

Deep Slow Breathing or Diaphragmatic breathing is the practice of breathing down deep into the abdomen, usually at a slow rate. Deep breaths mean the diaphragm muscle is free to press down and move viscera around making space for the lungs to expand.

There are several reasons why this can be difficult and restricted.

Tension in the abdominal muscles or the lower back will brace the viscera making it harder for the diaphragm muscle to move down and open the space for lungs to expand. I have found that MOST abdominal tension is emotional in origin. Emotions, such as fear, anger or dread create an instinctive and chronic state of abdominal tension; in fact, becoming aware of your abdominal state is a great way to begin to take control of your emotional state. Abdominal tension can also be due to habitual holding, scar tissue or shortened muscles created by sitting for hours each day

Tension in the lower back is typically the result of poor posture or, bracing due to lower back pain. It is ironic that this bracing, or guarding, was initially intended to protect the back and prevent further damage, because without movement, the lumbar area becomes dry and unhealthy, leading to a vicious downward spiral of pain, tension and deterioration. Is poor posture the cause or the effect of pain? Yes.

When faced with pain, whether mental anguish or simple physical hurt; I have a simple answer, movement and breathing are life.

Tummy ache, occasionally abdominal pain from cramps or poor digestive health can create abdominal tension, although it is always worth considering whether the tension is helpful or harmful...perhaps relaxing your abdomen will ease the pain and pressure in your tummy.

Many people wear clothing that is so tight that it literally restricts the abdominal region, creating a smaller available space for breathing.

Consider the ill effects of poor breathing habits:

Chronic Sympathetic Nervous System (fight, flight or freeze) dominant state, fatigue, low vitality and energy, sore upper body, frozen EMOTIONS

I find it fascinating that belly breathing is sometimes seen as unattractive given the implications of breathing high in the chest.

Our posture has a direct impact on the space available for respiration. When we stand hunched over or sit slumped in a chair our breathing is compromised. I don't think this information will surprise anyone but, the severity of the restriction and the consequences of poor breathing habits should alarm you enough to make a change or at the very least investigate for yourself the benefits of proper breathing.

Our lungs reside in a protective cage. The ribs and the musculature surrounding protect these vital organs from damage. Still, a cage is a cage and whether through loss of mobility in the rib structure and spine or constriction from tension in the muscles involved with breathing, we can find ourselves with diminished capacity or volume available for breath.

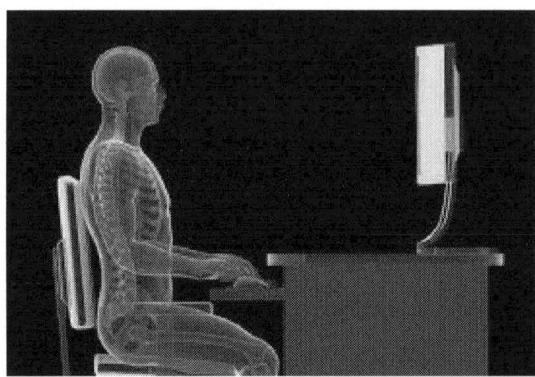

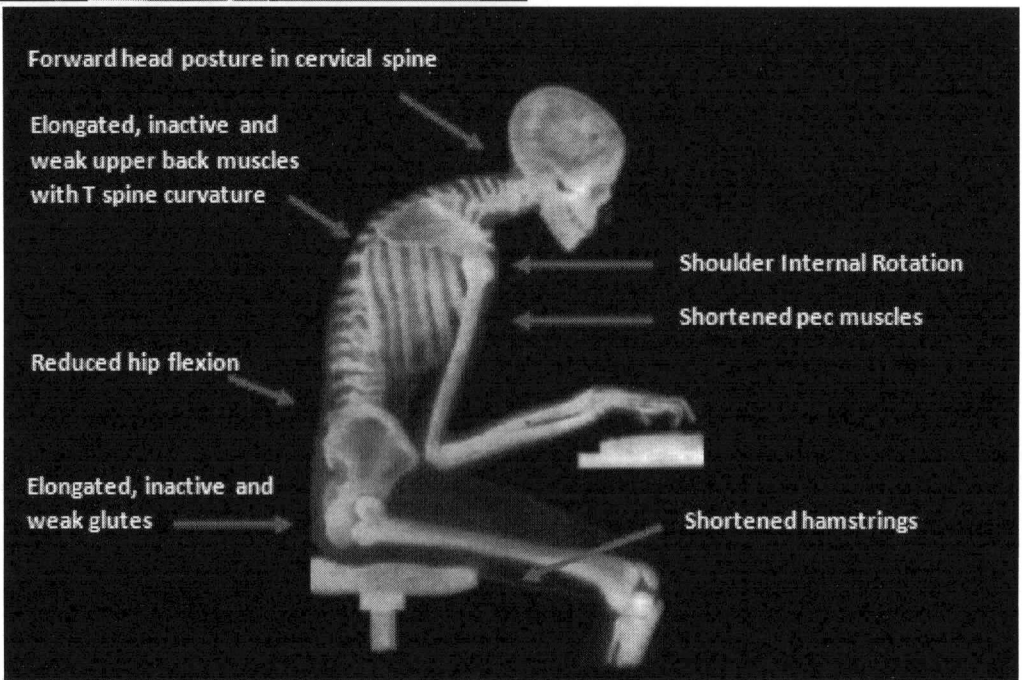

It is easy to see that in the second picture there is virtually no space for the lungs to expand into.

Standing and sitting with good posture is vital for easy, full breaths. There is another less obvious problem with poor posture. Poor posture creates muscular tension in the very muscles we use to breathe. If you consider that when our posture is correct our bones are aligned to structurally deal with the force of gravity. When we are out of alignment the muscles are forced to constantly work against the force pulling us down. And simple physics tells us that the long lever increases the downward force exponentially.

The bottom line is poor posture equates to poor breathing capability. So, how do we correct posture?

There are many exercises you can find to correct the muscular imbalances created by habitual poor posture. In this very book the breathing exercises will all help correct the residual effects of poor posture. Stretches to lengthen the shortened muscles and strengthening exercises to tone and neurologically awaken the weak and elongated muscles. I find that these exercises are useless without the collateral development of a psychological state that expresses as good posture.

So how can we learn to soften the belly and breathe properly for relaxed circumstances?

The act of diaphragmatic breathing itself will soften the belly.

It is that simple but, here are several additional ways to reduce abdominal tension:

Eat slower and consume less

Gentle stomach massage

Maintain digestive health

Keep psoas muscles in proper condition (don't sit so much)

Cat Cow stretch with wag the tail

Using the inhale to gently mobilize the spine

DRILL

Stand or sit quietly with good posture and allow the belly to soften while breathing, observe the swell of lower torso on inhale and the return to neutral on exhale. Repeat this exercise for as long as you are comfortable.

*about 10 minutes into this deep slow breathing you will feel the shifting into a parasympathetic nervous system (rest, recover and digest) dominant state

Beyond the belly

We can inhale and see our belly rise and swell. We can exhale and watch the belly fall. You can place a string around your chest and inhale and witness the expanding rib cage and observe as it relaxes back to a neutral position. Beyond this, we can, if we care to look, see and feel our lower back and kidney area swell out on the inhale, and feel *something* moving under the muscles and bone of the mid and upper thoracic region of the back. If we are sensitive to small movements, we can notice the movement of the scalene and trapezius muscles as we breathe in and out. Most of us can accept this idea that the experience of breathing can be felt throughout the torso at least. But what about the arms and legs and neck? Can we feel the effects of breathing there?

Absolutely.

A simple way to illustrate that the whole body is involved in the breathing process is:

DRILL

Lie down comfortably and breath normally for three inhale/ exhale cycles...on your third exhale, slowly expel as much air from your lungs as is possible, really try and empty them. You will see that the entire body is in contraction, even hands and toes. As you relax and then inhale the body will relax out into its normal condition. This exaggerated exhale vividly illustrates the whole body is engaged in the breathing process.

Air may not move through the knee joints, but if you are relaxed and pay close attention you can see the movement that is created there with each respiratory cycle. We can begin with the legs.

Lie down on your back and breathe gently and slowly into you lower abdomen. Recall that each inhale has a roundness, not just a hemisphere of movement. You will notice that the lower back or lumbar region descends slightly as you inhale. As the lower back moves down notice that the knees tend to lift or feel light. This is simple to explain; the lumbar spine is attached to the psoas muscles.

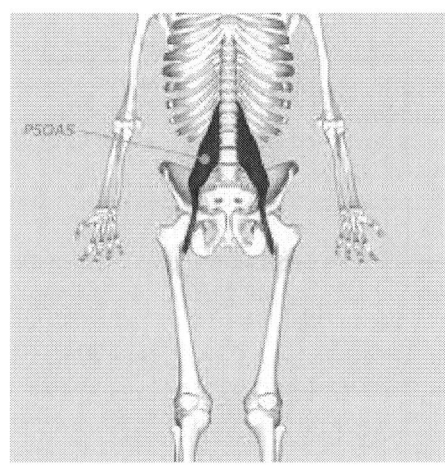

The psoas muscles extend down through the pelvic girdle and attach to the femur bones. As we inhale, and the spine moves slightly down, the psoas muscles pull upwards on the femurs creating slight upwards movement in the knees. Because our heels are in contact with the ground, as the knees move slightly upwards they exert a pulling on the heels creating a very slight ankle flexion.... this movement in the ankle changes the tension on the bottom of the foot which is transmitted through the plantar fascia creating movement all the way down even unto our toes.

Done properly, breathing can gently move and stretch the entire body.

And what of the arms?

As you inhale into the upper lobes of the lungs the pectoral muscles, the trapezius and rhomboid muscles, all the muscles in the upper torso are expanded and moved. The muscles wrap and connect with deltoid muscles and move the shoulder joints creating movement in the humerus bone, and all muscles and joints downstream in the arms.

It really is true; the whole body breathes. When we have tension, imbalance or poor posture, whether created by emotion or habitual activity and thought patterns, our breathing IS effected. And, conversely, our breathing directly impacts our entire body, including emotion, posture, thoughts and physiological condition.

Drill

To experience the whole-body during breath.

Lie down comfortably and begin deep and slow belly breathing.

Do not rush the diaphragmatic breathing...notice the expansion of the lower back area.

As you continue allow the breath to lengthen and fill up higher in the torso until you are breathing the wave breath, first the belly rises and then the chest, and then emptying from the top down.

This is breathing to explore the torso space.

Once you have achieved a level of comfort with this type of breath we will add legs and arms.

Breathe into the lower abdomen, bring your awareness to the slight movement of the lumbar spine.

As the lumbar spine relaxes and is gently pressed towards the floor or ground you may feel a lightening or lifting of your knees. What is happening is this. Your psoas muscles attach to your lumbar spine and run down through your pelvis and attach to your femur bones. Because we sit in chairs so much, most people have shortened psoas muscles. When your lumbar moves slightly downwards, your femur bones will be pulled upwards ever so slightly. This muscle that connects your spine to your legs will be your tactile target…your guide in a sense to breathing into your lower limbs. On the slow gentle inhale, feel the lumbar move, feel how this impacts the femur bones. Locate with your awareness (use hands if you need to) your psoas muscles. Allow your inhale, or more precisely your awareness, to travel down the psoas muscles into the femurs as you inhale. If you have room left, you can continue your inhale and breathe all the way down into your feet. Easy places to check in are the popliteal or behind the knees and just above the ankles on the back parts of your calves or soleus muscles. I find that wiggling the toes gently gives a great target for the awareness and helps get that awareness or breath all the way down to the toes.

Continue breathing down into the legs for several breath cycles at least, the longer the better.

Moving our attention up to the upper torso and the shoulders and arms, we will employ the same strategy of locating a muscle or a line of tension, to which we can attach our awareness and breathe along this tangible pathway until we can breathe directly into our arms and hands.

Modern culture is to spend hours hunched over a machine of some sort. Be it cellphone or keyboard, we spend hours with our shoulders rolled forwards and upper torso rounded. With the exception of gymnasts and dancers most of the people I see have really poor posture. We create shortened pectoral muscles and weak over stretched back muscles. This gives us an easy to locate line of tension.

Still lying flat on your back, lay your arms out from your body at a 45-degree angle palms up.

Consider first that your left lung has two lobes or sections and that your right lung has three lobes. Let's begin with the left side. Breathe into the upper lobe of the left lung, feel the expansion underneath the left pectoral muscle. Feel the pectoral muscles insertion and how they work with the shoulder joint.

The subclavius muscle is particularly good to be aware of while doing your inhale. As we inhale into the upper lobe of the lung there is movement in all the breathing muscles and the collarbone, this connection with the deltoid muscles, the latissimus dorsi muscles and the triceps muscles gives us the line of tension or the line of shortened muscles to use as our tactile target for our awareness driven by breath. Follow this line and its spiral down into the arm. Wiggle the finger as you continue to inhale and voila, you are breathing down, into your fingertips. Repeat the process on the other side and we have covered all the parts of the body. All that remains is to connect them and feel the breath move every part of your body.

Breathing to stretch and clean torso of tension

DRILL

Begin by lying on your back in a comfortable place. Relax and let your palms face the sky, leave space between your arms and your torso.

Breathe into the lower abdomen feeling the roundness of the breath. The stomach will softly rise, but also you will feel the lower back move gently outward as well. Stay with this type of breathing for three or four breath cycles, more if you desire.

Move up into the chest with the breath, feel the ribcage gently expand on the inhale and release back to a smaller size on the exhale. Three or 4 breaths here should be about right.

Next place one hand behind your head, as if you were lying on the grass looking up at the stars at night. Place your other hand on the rib cage under the arm that is behind your head. Slightly curve your body to open that side of the ribcage slightly more. Inhale gently into your hand, feel the space between the ribs, the intercostal muscles, gently stretch.

It is very important that you do not over stretch the intercostal muscles, be gentle, it's good to increase your ribcage's mobility and keep good blood flow to these muscles but stretch too far and you can have an intercostal muscle strain and that will slow down your recovery.

As you breathe into the open area try and move the breath around. Breathe down to the bottom of the lung, breathe into the back of the ribcage, back where they connect to the spine. breathe into the armpit area. Breathe underneath the shoulder blade. Explore and be playful with the breath, allowing it to roam around and wash the area of tension. Breath and awareness are very closely related in this exercise.

Change your arms and your body position and repeat the exercise on the other side of your body.

This is the beginning of cleaning the torso of tension.

After performing the previous exercise, you are ready to try a very interesting breathing practice. I will refer to it here as clearing the torso, but this exercise is one of the most powerful breathing practices available to you for a host of other reasons. I will leave you to discover these other benefits on your own. I believe sometimes it is better to allow a person to discover rather than to fill them with expectation.

BOTTOM TO TOP

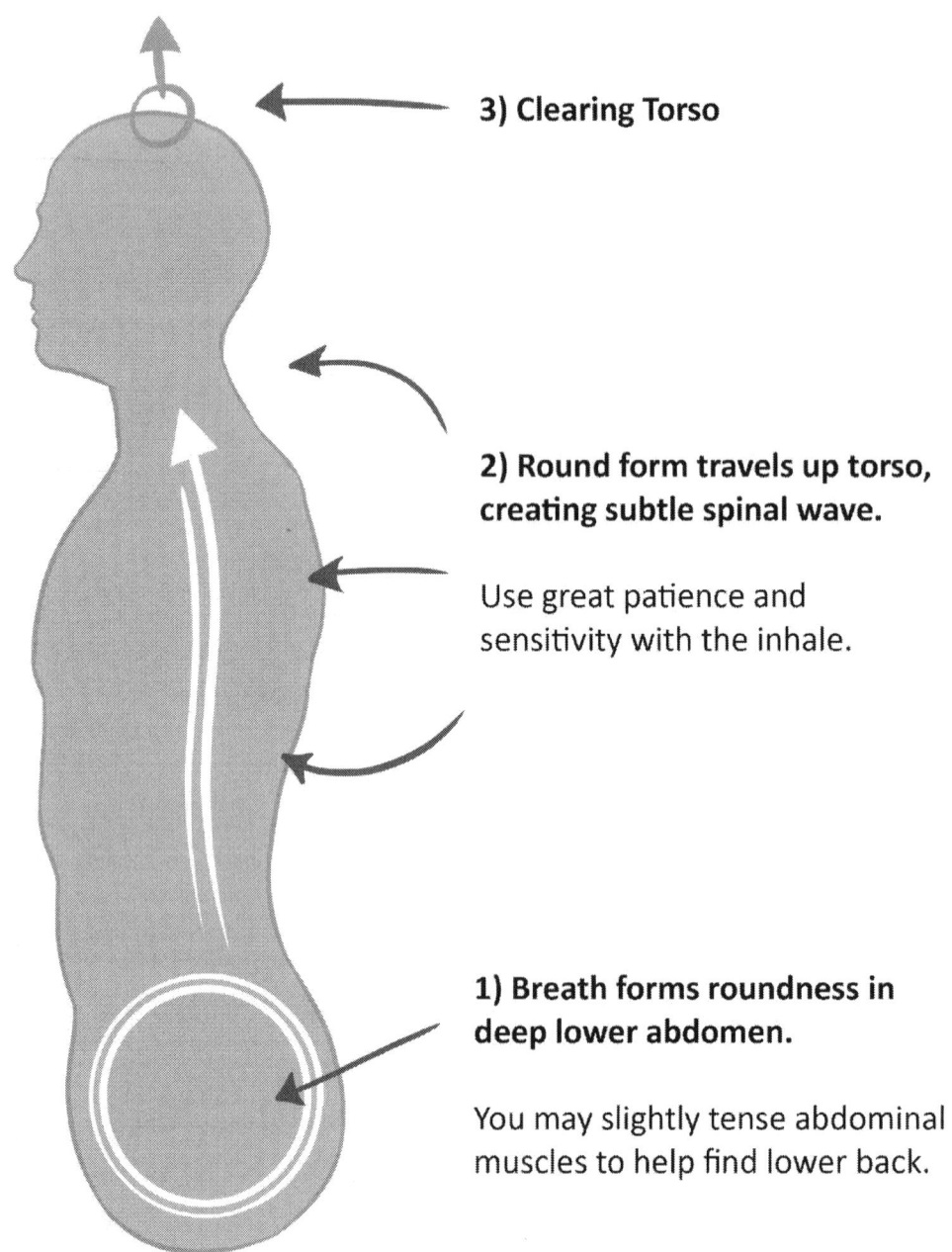

3) Clearing Torso

2) Round form travels up torso, creating subtle spinal wave.

Use great patience and sensitivity with the inhale.

1) Breath forms roundness in deep lower abdomen.

You may slightly tense abdominal muscles to help find lower back.

DRILL

Begin as before, lying down on your back, arms comfortably placed away from your torso palms up. You should be feeling relaxed from the previous exercise so don't press or strain, just allow the breath to work its magic for you.

Locate the space below the diaphragm muscle and above the perineum. Gently breathe down deep into this space, pay attention and feel the roundness created by the inhale. Be aware of the lower back as well as your lower abdomen.

I will describe two methods for the next step.

Method One:

Breathe gently but keep going into the lower abdomen. When you feel some volume there you can stop the inhale. Pull up on the perineum and slightly tense your muscles from the lowest part of your torso, slowly up the lower abdomen. Some people have said it is like rolling a tube of toothpaste from the bottom. As you introduce tension from the perineum up, you will feel the round volume of breath pressed up and moving up through your torso, up through the diaphragm area, up through the heart and lungs, traveling up the cylinder of your torso and continuing upwards through the throat and neck, even up through the head and out the crown.

Method 2:

This is much like the preceding method but requires much greater sensitivity. As you breathe softly but really deeply into the roundness of your lower torso area, allow your attention to notice the lower spine, even as low as the sacrum. As you begin to fill the space in the lower torso you will feel a slight pressure moving the lower vertebrae slightly down one by one in an ascending wave, you may slightly tense the abdominal muscles to increase the pressure on the spine but truly it is very subtle and slight. As you feel the lumbar begin to move begin to exhale and feel the spinal wave express all the way up lumbar, thoracic and cervical spine, finally expressing out the crown of the head.

This exercise is one of my personal favorites, but it does require some sensitivity and practice. Enjoy!

Awareness Breathing

I think it is contemporary culture to study the outside of our bodies, looking into a mirror or more often some other person's eyes to see who we are rather than developing an eye to see inside ourselves both physically and psychologically. There is good information to be garnered from our appearance, but the often-unexplored inner universe is even more rich and internal work lends itself to the healing of wounds and traumas un-seeable.

Proprioception is the awareness of the body in space and its orientation in relation to other objects and parts of itself. This might include body size and contour and awareness of internal processes such as heartbeat and digestives function. True self-awareness is more comprehensive, more all-encompassing than this, but is difficult to define. We can only move in the direction of more.

The question then becomes, how do we develop this self-awareness?

Awareness breathing is an exercise designed to foster and create awareness of the deep connection between your mind and your body. Awareness of this connection will enable you to manipulate and direct the inner functions of the body, enabling faster healing. As a side benefit you will have more vitality and energy as you reduce the effects of stress. There is an old saying, "mind over matter." The truth of this statement has never been more clear. To a large degree, you create your experience through perception and interpretation. It is increasingly clear that the body is as much a constituent of the mind as is the brain. This drill will help you map the body so that you can begin to work through it to create the experience you choose.

DRILL

This will be a visualization process; the more exact you can be with your focal point and its movement, the more benefit you will receive from this particular exercise.
I myself use the image of a tiny, microscopic-sized spaceship shaped something like a stingray fish; my ship is chrome and flies very well. You may choose any device you wish. Some children I have taught this method prefer planes or butterflies as their flying focal points. It doesn't matter what you choose, but it definitely matters that you *do* choose as specifically as you can.
Begin by lying down in a comfortable space, a warm floor or a hospital bed, it doesn't matter. It need only be a place to relax as deeply as you can.
If possible, turn your palms up toward the sky.

Feel the length of your spine, particularly the cervical spine or neck region.

Just observe your breath going in and out. Your stomach rises on the inhale and falls on the exhale. Don't rush, this is not an exercise for technique. This is to develop awareness. As you begin the exercise your inhale will be light and soft, a tendril rather than a torrent. Your exhale should be relaxed, *poof,* like a soap bubble bursting, all tension in the body gone with the exhale. It may help to form the sound *Ha* or *huh* in your throat.

Inhale your spaceship in through the nose, spiraling up into the sinus cavity and swirling out into the grey matter of your brain. As you fly through the actual meat that is inside your skull feel it relax and soften everywhere you fly your awareness. Be as specific as possible with the location of your ship. Is it swirling or looping, tracing figure eights or circles, in the middle or near the outside? The more specific the better. Fly through the brain on the inhale, *poof!* release all tension in the body on the exhale and repeat three or four times or until you can feel the brain matter relaxing. The volume of breath will be fairly small at this point; do not allow your inhale to increase your tension any more than you have to. When you are doing this part of the exercise correctly, it feels as if you can map your own brain, literally feeling the different areas and parts of the whole.

Next, continue to breathe through the grey matter but now go a little deeper, down into the base of the brain, the hindbrain and deeper into the medulla oblongata. The place where the spinal cord and the brain connect, the primitive part of the brain. Be specific with your awareness and gentle with your breath; still swirling down, still *poof!* exhale and release tension. Please repeat this through the brain and down deeper into the brain stem several times. Often you will observe that a person who is doing this exercise will slightly tuck their chin, elongating the cervical spine, lengthening the neck.

Next, continue through the brain and brain stem, deeper now. The breath will emerge onto the interior surface of the spine, meaning *not* inside the spinal column, but on its surface facing the inside of the body. The breath is still soft and light but there will be slightly more volume now. Inhale down, deeper, following the spine until you reach the level of the heart muscle. Now, curve out from the spine and swirl through, swoop through, the heart muscle itself. Don't rush. Stay calm and relaxed and feel the breath, the awareness, your spaceship flying through the muscle, relaxing the heart itself. The chest will soften and relax and open; for some people, this can be a very emotional place. It is absolutely amazing how our physiology and our emotion relate. Spend as much time here as you would like. There is no rush. It is *your* exercise, your awareness and your experience. Inhale down, exhale "huh" and release tension.

Next, continue as before, breathing through the brain, brain stem, swirling out through the heart and then:

Allow the breath to return to the interior surface of the spine and travel downward, up the slope of the lumbar region, then swooping down as you follow the contours of the spine to the sacrum; even deeper following the curve of the tailbone and swirling back upward into the lower abdomen. Fly your awareness as you wish, looping and swirling and dancing through the lower abdomen. For me it is reminiscent of the middle school drawings of electron orbits, light doing loop the loops and infinity signs all through my lower torso.

By this time, the volume of air you are inhaling will be large. Still, bring it in gently and lightly and stay precise with your focus. Your exhale will not be as quick as it was earlier; even relaxing as completely as you can it will take a little longer to travel out of your body.

On the inhale, you should feel the connection between your nose and the crown of your head all the way down your spine to your tailbone and up into your soft, relaxed belly.

This is truly a beautiful exercise when done properly. You can stay with this exercise for as long as you want or for only a few minutes.

TOP TO BOTTOM

"Awareness" breathing for the torso space

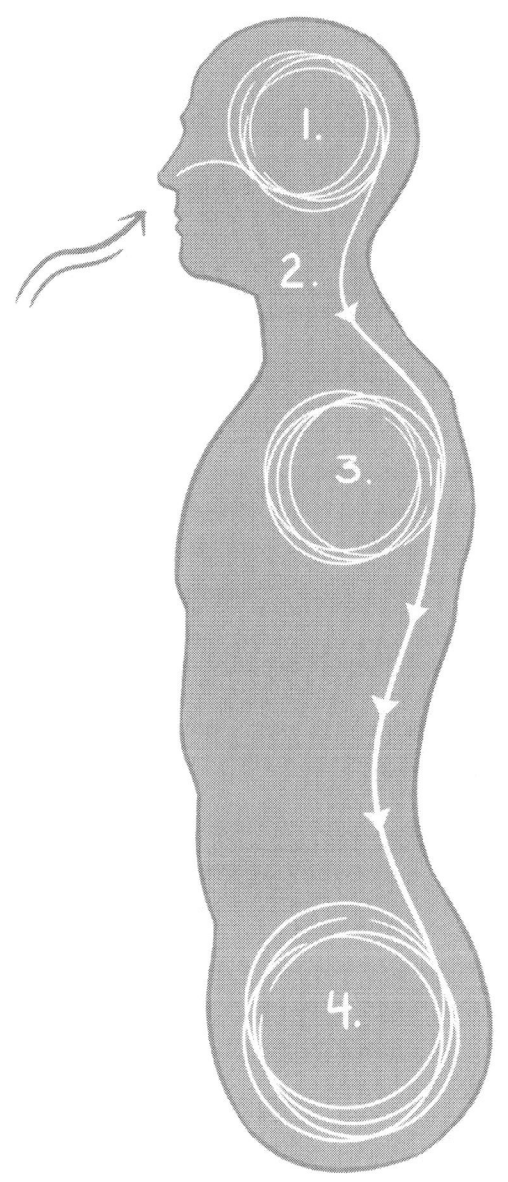

INHALE
Light, thin, soft.
This is not a volume breath.

EXHALE
Poof, like a soap bubble bursting.

1) Relax brain
2) Brain stem
3) Heart
4) Lower abdomen

Breath travels on interior surface of the spine.

Stretching the Body (Pandiculation)

DRILL

Picture a cat stretching as it rises from a nap. Yawning and stretching its facial muscles and flexing the muscles in its cat body while moving it's spine and splaying it's toes wide.

Lying on your back spread your body out like a giant letter X or a humongous starfish.

This exercise should feel as if you are just waking up, luxuriate in having a body to inhabit, be a little lazy and slow and in no hurry to arise from the warm bed.

As you inhale, expand your limbs and torso and become as large as you possibly can. You will notice that this will create a small amount of tension in the muscles. This is good to work with.

Inhale and expand your shape and simultaneously wiggle your fingers and your toes. Repeat this several times.

Inhale and expand and circle your wrists and your ankles, exhale and relax.

Inhale slowly and move your shoulders. Rotate them internally and externally. Take the time to relish the movement. Exhale and relax completely.

Inhale and expand and slowly undulate your spine, maintaining a slight tension in your entire body, then exhale and relax.

Inhale and expand your shape as large as you possibly can and then begin small undulations throughout your entire body. Express waves down and up and from the center out, do not hold your breath. Make these movements gentle and slow, with some minimum amount of tension to help you remain aware of as many muscles as possible. Feel how your body's shape and silhouette change. Repeat several times.

Now, make your body as long as you possibly can, stretching your arms up overhead and pointing your toes downward, like an Olympic diver.

Inhale, stretch and reach, elongate your body and have slight tension, flex your ankles, pointing your toes up, then down again and sigh out your exhale. Repeat several times.

Now, make your body as wide as you can.

Inhale and stretch your arms as wide as you can reach, open your palms wide. **Remember, do not hold your breath**. The inhale should feel as if it is creating the expansion in your body. When your inhale stops, your expansion will stop, and you will begin your exhale and relax.

Continue to reach wide on the inhales and flex your wrists, point up as if you were pressing two walls away from your body. Point down and press. Explore different movements of the wrists.

If your health allows it you can turn on your sides or even your stomach and try these," inhale and expand and move your extremities". The contact with the floor or the bed will create tactile sensation and send information to your brain.

All these movements contribute to proprioception, knowing the size, shape and location in space of your body. And by linking the breathing to the expanding and moving you will be very aware of your internal expansion and movement of muscles involved in breathing.

As you become comfortable with the expansion and contraction we will add the element of stretching.

DRILL

Exhale stretches

Lie comfortably on you back. Inhale and feel your arms and legs reach out as far as you can. Open your palms from their center as open as you possibly can. Press the backs of your hands down into the floor as if to stick them there or glue them in that location, glue your heels to the floor as well.

Now, as you exhale, do not allow your hands or your feet to contract and move back towards your center. As you continue to exhale you will feel a very strong pulling sensation in your connective tissues. As you exhale your torso will be shrinking and this will pull from the center of your body, stretching your limbs quite intensely!

After five or six exhale stretches stop, relax and notice how much more open your joints and your limbs feel.

Natural People or Standing Breathwork

I met Professor Teng Ying Bo in Beijing, China. He is a small man but exudes an enormous and deep sense of calm and health. I have never seen him tired or slow, he is so full of good energy that he seems to glow from within. I met him in Fragrant Hills Park and he delivered my second qigong lesson of the day. Healing my broken leg was the first magical thing I witnessed/ experienced Professor Teng accomplish. He practices in Thailand and China and if you have the means to go train with him, I highly recommend that you do so.

Professor Teng is a genuine master of qigong and he has the same traits that all the Masters I have met demonstrate.

In my lifetime, I have met, in person, five Masters. Some folks ask right away, what is a Master? I can say that you will know one when you meet. These people have mastered their various arts and practices to a degree that allows the hard-won wisdom they earned via their individual practices to have universal applicability. These people have, by virtue of mastering their art, gained a wisdom and a perspective that serves in all of life's travails.

These Masters have several things in common. It goes without saying that they are the pinnacle, the peak expression of the art that they practice but, in addition, the masters all exhibit a profound patience. When they interact with seekers they do not feel any compulsion to entertain, only to transfer the knowledge they have.

Vladimir Vasiliev, Teng Ying Bo, Fong Ha, Master Yu of Huashan and one other un-named Taoist adept from China, these people have taught me that there really is no secret or shortcut. Any secret is only made so by the students' refusal to actually follow the teacher's straight forward wisdom.

Professor Teng on the very first day I met him asked me to stand still and breathe for one hour. He was unapologetic, in fact he was, it seems to me, wholly unmoved by me in any way. But I, I was moved by him without question, shored up and given a lift on his enormous and generous wave of energy. I will share the first and the simplest breathwork that he shared with me. I give him all credit. And I encourage you to seek him out and train with this man if at all possible. He IS a true master of qigong and breathwork. While the exercise I will share with you here is simple, do not be deceived, it has a fundamental power that will absolutely change you as a being IF you practice as Professor Teng presents it.

Standing Breath Exploration

NOTE

The following four drills are best done in order and consecutively. It is possible to break them out and practice each individually, but I do not recommend it.

DRILL

Begin by choosing a suitable location, at a minimum it should be safe and somewhat discrete. People do not know what to make of a person standing still, doing nothing except breathing. One exception is China, where if you begin your practice before sunup you may be surprised to find people joining you in practice or even applauding and smiling and wanting to know you when you are done.

Optimally the location you choose will be a natural space, Mountains, oceans, streams and trees, deserts all have their own unique energies and you will be infused with these energies to some degree.

If no good natural space is available to you don't be deterred. You can practice indoors with a window cracked and still enjoy amazing results.

Start with your feet parallel and hip or shoulder width apart.

Lift your toes and create a good arch, feel the feet and how they rest upon the earth or floor. Massage the feet a bit by leaning forwards, backwards and side to side. Gently come to stasis and let your toes relax back and lightly rest on the ground.

Relax the knees, soften the knees so that the knee caps are released down, maintain a slight bend in the knees so blood can flow easily. I have personally witnessed people pass out from standing too long with their knees locked. You can be seriously injured, so please DO NOT LOCK the knees.

Release the hips. This is more releasing the lower back, but the easiest place to check for tension is in the hips. You should feel that if a butterfly landed on your hip it would create a wave of movement. That is relaxed.

Drop the shoulders, release tension from the trapezius muscles and lift the crown towards the heavens.

Often when we say relax the shoulders we really need to raise the crown of the head towards the sky. The feeling is as a string of pearls dangling, *suspended from the heavens*, with space between every vertebra.

Arms should be hanging loose and natural by the sides.

Master Fong Ha would issue these instructions to get you standing in a natural, loose way and then he would leave you there for some 45 minutes or more, allowing you to find the most comfortable and therefor most correct way of standing.

You will feel some discomfort as time passes, shift your weight or make micro adjustments to your position to get yourself comfortable and try and breathe through the areas of discomfort.

One interesting note is that when I see people standing perfectly stable, I know they are not releasing as much tension as possible. When you are truly seeking and releasing tension, it is as if you are trying to stack your bones one atop the other using no muscle or as little muscle as is possible.

This is an inherently dynamic and unstable posture, in fact, every heart beat changes your center of gravity, every breath changes your center of gravity so there will definitely be movement with your still stance. Further into your standing, muscles located deep within the body, generally inaccessible to our conscious mind, will begin to release and let go. On occasion you may experience a sudden almost violent shift in of the body as you release deeper and deeper into looseness and freedom.

Having achieved this stance, it is time to begin the deeper training.

DRILL

Begin by starting at the top of the head, the crown and the scalp, release tension there. Take your time spending a minimum of three breaths letting go of excess muscle contraction. Some areas will require several minutes to truly release. You know your body, or you will, so don't rush. Take your time and piece by piece move down through the body relaxing as deeply as you can.

Scalp, face, eyes, tongue, throat, neck, trapezius, shoulders, arms, elbows, forearms, hands, upper back and chest, middle back and upper abdomen, lower back and lower abdomen, hips and gluteal muscles, relax the whole pelvic area. Move down into the legs, thighs, knees, lower legs, ankles and feet,

As you move through the body it will be a constant adjusting and re-releasing of parts as you work to maintain balance and the standing position while simultaneously relaxing as deeply as you can. Don't give up and don't rush. The less tension you have in your body the more productive the breathwork and energy work will be. You are preparing for some magic so be thorough.

Once you have achieved a deep level of relaxation and quiet it is time to begin the 5 different qigong postures I will be sharing in this chapter.

Heaven, Earth, Man

DRILL

Standing naturally move the arms out to your side just enough to allow air to touch all the arm pit. The idea is to have a pea sized space under the arms.

Located on the crown of your head is a point where energy can move into or escape from the body easily. This point is known as the baihui point. Use your awareness and as you inhale "breathe" Yang energy from the heavens down through this point, straight through the torso and into the lower abdomen, or lower tantien (dantien). Continue this inhale configuration for as long as you like but a minimum of 9 unhurried breath cycles is recommended. Inhale down through your crown into your lower abdomen, exhale and relax the whole body more completely.

Next, inhale Yin energy from the Earth up through the yongquan or bubbling well point, located on the soles of your feet just behind the ball of the foot and in the center. The two streams of breath, awareness, energy, travel up the legs and into the lower dantien (tantien) or lower abdomen. Again, a minimum of 9 cycles is recommended but you may continue for as long as you wish.

For our purposes, Yang energy is considered spiritual in nature and Yin energy is considered nurturing and healing in nature. Both energies are spiritual and both energies are healing in their own way. We are focusing on awareness. Inhale Yin energy up through the bubbling wells, through the legs and into the lower abdomen. Exhale and relax and let go even more tension.

Finally, inhale Yang energy from the Heavens and Yin energy from the Earth simultaneously. The three streams of energy or awareness meeting and mingling/mixing in the lower abdomen or lower dantien.

Balanced between these energies is human.

Inhale Yang down through the crown and Yin up through the feet at the same time. Exhale and surrender more tension. Maintain this breathwork for as long as you like, but a minimum of 9 breath cycles is recommended. Often it will feel as if you are standing on the very peak of a mountain, waist deep in snow, feeling the open space and sky above and around you, while experiencing the rooted feeling of being connected with the earth through the mountain.

Clean the meridians

Second posture from Professor Teng Ying Bo's standing series.

After the standing and inhaling Yang energy from the Heavens and Yin energy from the earth and then relaxing deeply on the exhale, you are ready to try the second posture and exercise.

DRILL

From the neutral standing position raise the arms slightly higher to the side. Allowing room enough for a grape or a small lemon under the arm in the arm pit area. You are creating the architecture for the breathing exercise which follows.

Bend the knees and slowly sing towards the earth, stopping when you feel tension in the quadriceps. For this exercise, we want to maintain a constant tension in the thighs.

Slowly rotate your forearms until your palms are facing behind you. Press your palms backwards as if you are standing against a wall and the palms stop even with the imaginary wall, roughly in the same plane as your back.

This is truly a working posture. I mean that in the sense that you will use your intention to DRIVE any stale or stagnant chi or energy out of your body, through your fingertips into the earth. As you inhale collect the stale and stagnant chi, as you exhale, drive the energy up, out and down through your fingertips. We keep tension in the thighs, so the energy does not travel back up through the legs. Often you will find yourself sweating profusely while performing this exercise.

I don't have a scientific, or rather a western based scientific explanation for why this occurs. I can only report that it does in fact work. The idea is that the Earth is like a good mother. She receives the tired, negative chi and like fertilizer, changes it so that it becomes a healthy Yin energy that nurtures and heals and grows.

In this section of the book I am using terms that seem fantastical or foreign to some of our western ideas. I too struggle with these words. But I cannot deny the reality of my own personal experience. If you try these exercises you WILL get results, regardless of how difficult it is to accept the terminology.

Sometimes it is wise to consider that this technology has been around for a very, very long time and has proven itself effective even if we do not understand why.

Exchange Essence Chi

When you have cleansed yourself with the Cleaning the meridians exercise, move directly into exchanging essence chi exercise.

DRILL

Allow the body to rise back to full standing, straightening the legs and moving upwards until the quadriceps relax. DO NOT LOCK THE KNEES! Remember the very, real danger of passing out if you lock the knees. Keep the knees soft, with kneecaps down and devoid of tension. Check in with your posture, making certain that you are lifting the crown and relaxing the hips down so that the spine is as a string of pearls dangling from the heavens. Relax the arms until there is just enough room in the armpits for air to contact all the skins surface. This is a return to the original natural standing.

In China the skin is sometimes referred to as the third lung. For the purpose of this next exercise we will be training our awareness and "breathing" through the pores of our skin.

As you stand, re-verify your deep state of relaxation. Balance your bones one atop the other so that gravity and connective tissue keep you aloft and upright in perfect long, tall posture. As little muscular tension as you can possibly manage and still remain standing. Recall that standing in this manner is inherently unstable and there should be very small or micro movements taking place at all times. If you are completely stable you are not relaxed enough. There is a distinct awareness of space between the joints, as if you can feel them opening and allowing the good synovial fluid to bathe the joint.

And, being to "inhale" through the pores of your skin. Slow deep breaths. "Exhale" through all the pores of your skin.

This is fascinating and occasionally dramatically beautiful exercise. First you will become acutely aware of your body's shape and size and displacement. This is followed by an awareness of some thermal layer that surrounds the body due to the heat being given off as your body processes occur. It is an eye opened for some folks, for the first time they experience that their skin is not a hard boundary, that many human attributes extend beyond the skin. Lastly, when you are truly successful with this exercise you will find that you are not really as distinct from your environment as you had perhaps believed. You will experience a sort of merging with your environment, or at the least an exchanging of essence chi with your environment.

So, standing naturally. Inhale essence chi from your environment and exhale your essence chi into the environment. There is an exchange of energy with your surroundings. It is best to do this exercise when you are in nature, some beautiful energy filled space such as a beach or mountain or desert. You can do this exercise with a tree or a plant as well.

Insignificance

After exchanging essence chi exercise, we will look at one more standing breathing exercise.

When you are ready to end your standing practice, perform the following exercise.

DRILL

Inhale into the very center of your being, keep the inhale thin and slow, filling the internal space from the center out. As your inhale fills the torso space, continue out into the limbs, the head, even beyond the boundary of the skin, expanding as far out as your awareness will allow.

Exhale and come back into the body, the torso, the center of your being-ness and smaller, until you experience yourself as a tiny insignificant speck, which soon winks completely out of existence.

Rest for a brief moment in this non-existence then resume breathing as you inhale as before.

Two rounds of this quieting breath are enough.

Occasionally people experience some worry that they may actually die when the breath ceases movement and awareness shrinks and is gone. To date that has not happened, and I expect that it never will.

Empathy Breathing

Science says that no consciousness exists in isolation. Our brains, our minds communicate without words, without visual confirmation. Our subconscious minds are always connecting and communicating. When you can't speak the depths of your worries or the love, you can still breath to empathy.

Our emotional state is deeply entwined with our breathing. When you understand this truth, you can begin to use breathing to understand How another person is feeling and to connect on a deeply human level with that other person.

It is best if you have some physical contact with the person you want to empathize with, touch alone is a profoundly connecting and communicating modality, but these exercises can be done at a distance if you are perceptive enough.

I have found two types of environments that work best for practicing breathing to empathy, but you can do the exercises anywhere. If you are indoors, try to find a comfortable but somewhat austere environment, with minimal distractions. Television, computers and cell phones make it more difficult to focus as do interruptions from people coming in and out. You work with what you have but quiet is better. If you are outdoors you need a safe place with not much wind. Heavy layers of clothing make these exercises more difficult but not overly so. Sounds such as bird calls and flowing water are pleasant and help a person relax.

DRILL

Begin by sitting or lying next to the person, sit back to back if side by side is too confrontational. Hold hands if the person has that sort of relationship with you. And again, sometimes the person will not want to engage with you at all and you will just work from a distance to understand how they feel.

To listen to another, you must turn down your own internal noise.

Calm yourself by breathing deep slow rhythmic breaths. Release excess tension and become aware of the physical connection between the two of you or the texture of the space separating you.

DRILL

Simultaneous breathing

Breathe together, simultaneously. As your partner inhales so do you, as they exhale so do you. Maintain this awareness and compliance with the other person's rhythm of breathing for as long as you wish. Two or more minutes is best, 5 minutes is even better. As you match the other's breathing you will begin to feel the other person's emotions and a process of entrainment can occur. If the other person is in distress you can begin to breathe just slightly more slowly, slightly more deeply and see if this draws the person with you. It is possible to lead a person out of distress, even to de-escalate a serious confrontation by empathizing, entraining and then leading with the breath to a place of more calm, more relaxation.

This is not a trick. Your nervous system must lead the movement towards a more serene, relaxed and stable state. Your breathing must first work on you and then you can assist the other person, like emergency oxygen masks in an airplane.

While leading another person towards a calmer emotional state is a nice practice it is not the primary purpose of empathetic breathing. The first and primary purpose of breathing to empathy is to **actually empathize** with another, experience and understand the feelings that they are immersed in. This can be painful, scary or sad. But by connecting you will be providing a profound service to the other person and you will be educating yourself as to how the other person feels.

DRILL

Complementary breathing

As your partner **inhales**, you **exhale**. As your partner **exhales**, you **inhale**. By participating in the same rhythm as your partner you will forge a very close connection. I find it even more intensely intimate than breathing simultaneously. Everything that is true about simultaneous breathing holds true for complementary breathing, but the connection is intensified. This type of breathing works particularly well if you are hugging or embracing the person you wish to connect with. You WILL feel them, and they will feel you.

When your intention is empathy, it becomes a powerful force for connection and intimacy. You are communicating to your partner that you desire connection, that they are not alone and that you wish to join them in their state, you wish to meet them where they are.

We as humans have a fervent need to be seen and known. Enjoy this beautiful exercise.

DRILL

Advanced Empathetic Breathwork

Sit back to back.

Practice breathing simultaneously, then complementary. Stay with this practice until you feel a deep sense of peace and connection to your partner.

Draw the breath in through your nose, up through your brain and down, down the brain stem, down the spine and out to swirl through your heart. Continue the slow inhale and bring it into your partner's heart through your backs. Allow your awareness to travel down into your most loving heart self and then continue through the skin, through the illusion of separateness and into your partners feeling, sensing center.

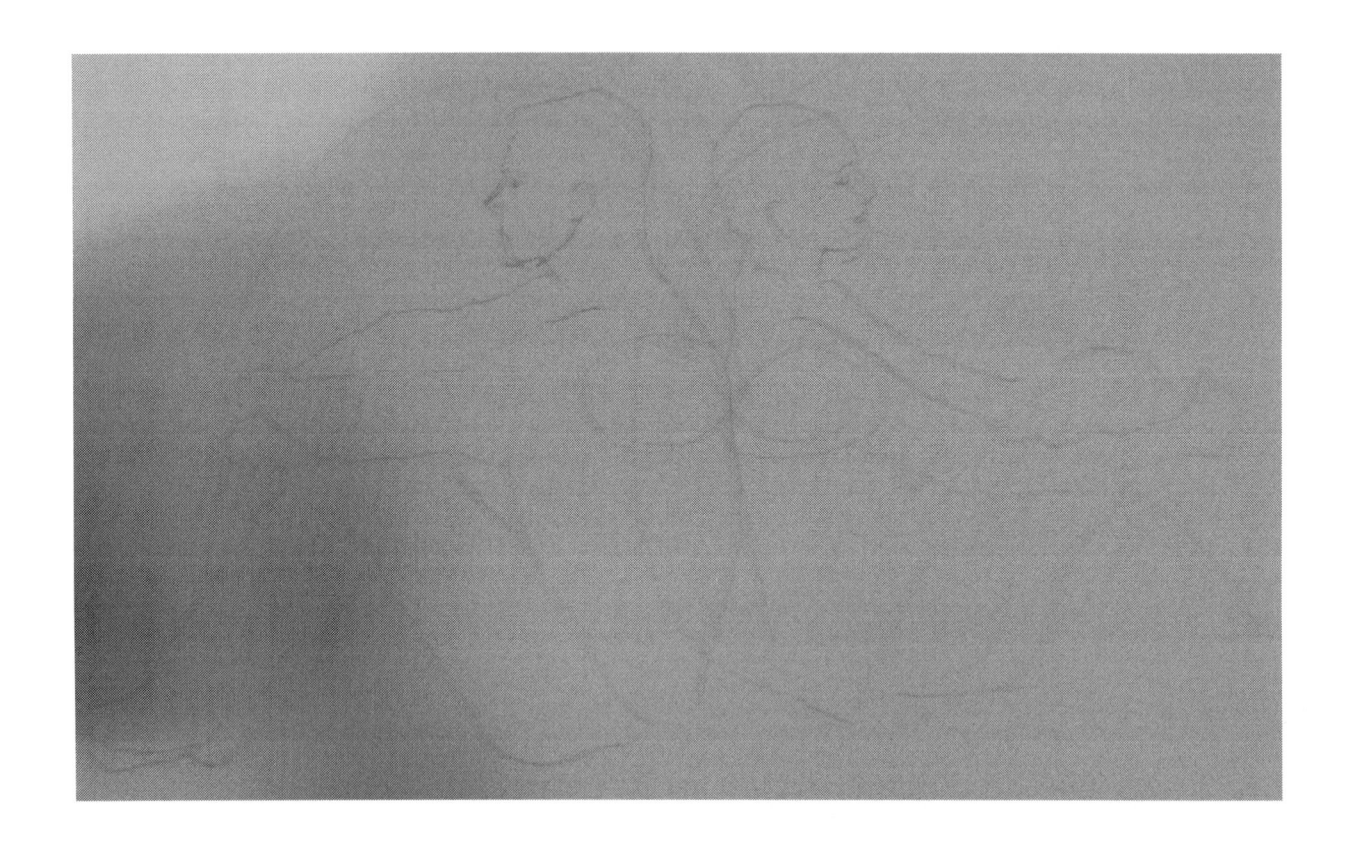

Bonus Material for Empathy:

Overwhelmed by the energetic noise of a city or an emotionally chaotic relationship? Stuck in a hospital room, sterile, your suffering a number on a chart and your sleep interrupted for blood draws? You may need respite from over stimulation, a break from the buzz.

DRILL

Experiencing insignificance

Pray, meditate and breathe.

Go to the ocean, stand or sit on the beach. Smell the salt air. Feel the breeze caress your skin. Taste the salt and the sea. Wade out into it if possible. Enjoy the waves rising and falling. Stare out as far as you can see into the vastness, feel the enormity and experience the bliss of insignificance.

Go to the desert or the mountains or the forest. Go anywhere where awe is the appropriate state.

The idea is to experience your place. You do not have to carry every feeling. The universe is large enough to hold all.

DRILL

Elemental Empathy

With the right mindset you can immerse your fingers in a glass of still water and connect to the ocean. You can touch the dirt in the pot of a plant and feel the majesty of a mountain. You can feel the warmth of the sun shining through a window and onto your skin and remember the cleanliness of the desert.

Empathize with nature. Nature can teach us how to hold all of the noise in proper perspective.

Note: Some people self-medicate using music. I am not a music expert, but it seems these are emotional immersions, meant to obliterate all but one emotion and that being one of the artist's choosing. I don't know enough to render any opinion I only want to point out that it is quite a different experience than the one to which I am referring you.

Breathing through the mind

After you are relaxed in the body. When you have some success with the Awareness Breathing exercise, you may wish to try the following:

DRILL

Remember some moment, some event from your life.

Recall the moment as clearly as you can.

Remember smells, sounds, tastes, body position and sensations.

Understand that this memory is a construct of the mind. The body and the brain are recreating the experience in hormonal and electrical ways.

Then simply begin to breathe through the memory, through the minds construct.

Observe as the memory fades like fog exposed to sunlight. Feel as the body returns to a relaxed calmness.

Your inhales are the same as in the Awareness Breathing exercise, your exhales are more complete, quicker and with just a bit more force behind them. Use your exhales to release all tension from your body and your mind.

After a few breaths, leave this exercise and just remain in the relaxed body. Enjoy the sensation of calm and rest.

When ready wiggle your finger and toes and bring your attention back to the external world. Relax, smile. Enjoy. You are a survivor.

BRAINSTORM

Working with Memories

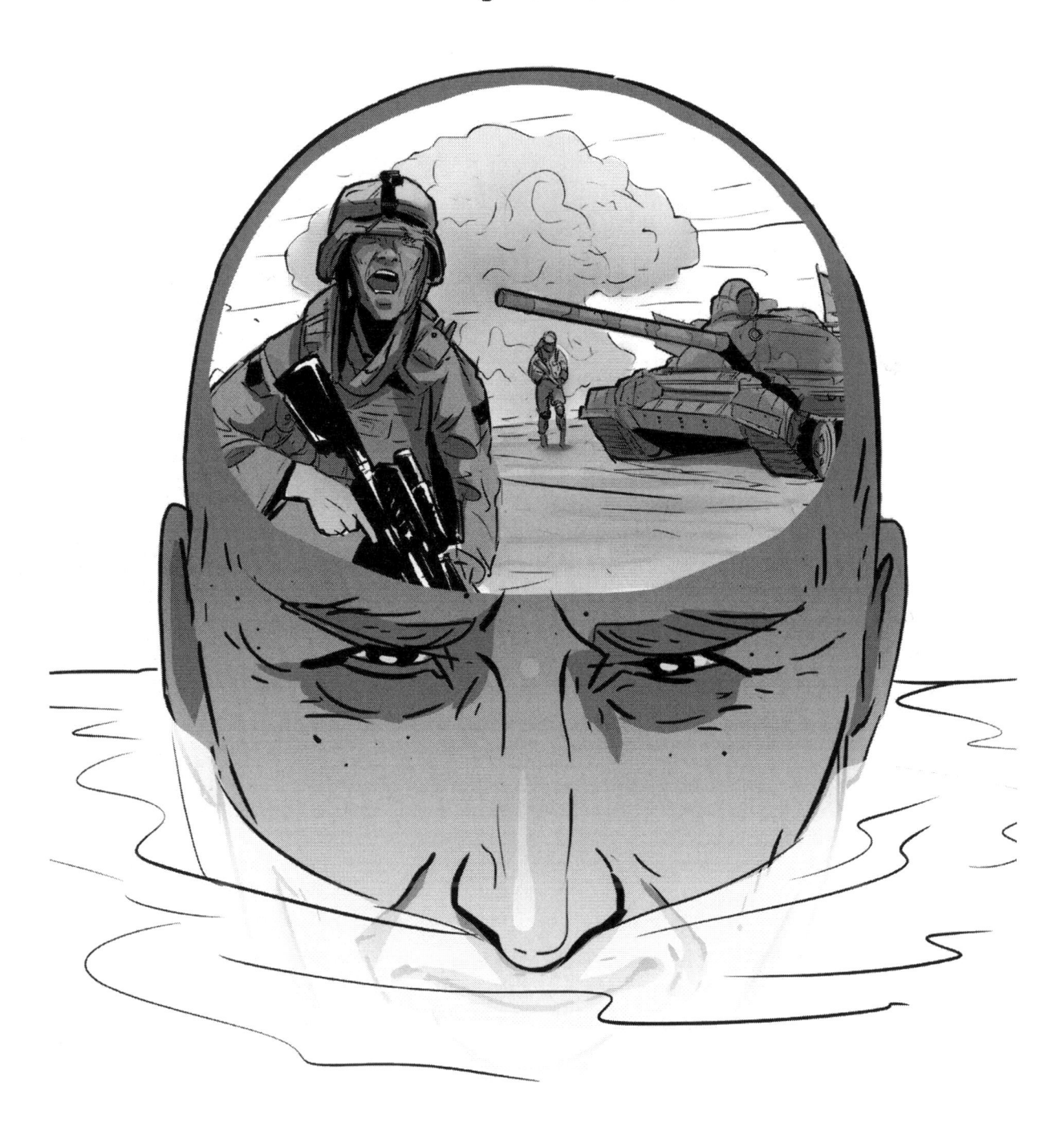

43

In One, Out One

Fall of 2008 I traveled to Toronto, Ontario, Canada to train with my teacher Vladimir Vasiliev. I had been training in Systema, or Russian Martial Art for several years and was certified as an instructor of Russian Martial Art by Vladimir. The topic of the seminar was breathwork.

During the years I had been training with Vladimir I had already been completely fascinated, captured and was hardcore about the breathing exercises he gave us. When I signed up to go to Toronto I was expecting more of the same type of exercise, similar yet mind blowing, just led by the man himself.

I am always reluctant to leave my family and my school. Financially it is a serious challenge for me to travel, so I am limited to only going to train when I consider it to be an essential training that cannot be missed. This was the situation in 2008 with the breathing seminar. At the time I don't think it was a super popular topic, but in my own progression I was certain it would be ground breaking. Secretly I imagined that some super-secret breathing technique would be taught that would revolutionize my training.

The seminar format was unusual to begin with in that it was three days of 6 hours a day training. And if my memory serves, there was a video link with another instructor from Moscow who specialized in the types of training we were to do.

For some length of time we sat and listened to various explanations and went through a few stretching and breathing exercises and then we were told to stand up and start walking around the room breathing in one step, out one step. In one step, out one step.

There were a few minor variations…. walk faster…slower…walking backwards was the big exciting break, but mainly we walked in a room sized circle for 6 hours breathing in one step out one step.

As hour after hour went by I felt disappointment building. I had never experienced disappointment in relation to Vladimir's teaching before, on the contrary, I was usually stunned by the depth and simplicity of his teachings. That evening I returned to the bed and breakfast where myself and a training partner were staying. It was a beautiful little room in a house on the same street as the Toronto Russian Orthodox Church, a truly lovely place. As we sat around preparing for sleep I hesitantly broached the subject. Is that it? Why couldn't we just do this at home. Why did I sale everything and leave my family to come way up here and walk in a circle and breathe? My friend, known as a trunk of the Systema tree expressed the same bewilderment? Well, we were here now; may as well go back the next day.

Day two, we came in and immediately the instruction was walk and breathe… in one, out one. Now backwards, now forwards slowly. My mind was full of complaint, frustration, regret, disappointment, disbelief…and then…nothing. I don't know what happened but suddenly my being was different. Arms swung in concert with legs moving and twisting the torso, air was moved in and out without tension. Thought ceased and I was immersed in this experience, this miracle of walking.

It's an unfamiliar feeling to be clean inside. To have the white noise that occupies my brain space, the constant internal conversation and measuring gone. A fascinating and primal state of awareness takes hold and all the little details the data that we ordinarily miss are unexpectedly available. The present moment has a wholeness to it. It is impossible to be surprised and it as if you can foresee future events, because you see the permutations and lines of causality that radiate out from every point. At the same time, past and future are almost oxymoron's…it is as if here and now is all that exists, and we are expanded to fill that space. I wonder if this is how our ancestors walked wild, surrounded by danger and yet they survived, even created art. I know that for myself I have experienced this type of uber view a few times spontaneously, one notable moment was the moment I was shot multiple times at close range. I had the same omniscient perspective and afterward the question always followed me, why are we not like this all the time?

I don't really remember the rest of the day now, so overwhelming was the sensation of being present that I don't truly remember the rest of that day. I do remember that we switched over to studying how to work against a person with a knife at some point and it was laughable. The seminar participants were split into two groups, half drew names from a hat and were supposed to go attempt to stab that person with a training knife. It wasn't much of a drill, because after those hours of breathing it was apparent who was going to try and stab you the moment they read your name on the tiny slip of paper. Generally, the intended "victim" would begin laughing and walk out of the room, to go get a drink or use the restroom, and their "attacker" would be left standing there forlorn with training knife in hand and nothing to do.

In one, out one. Walk and breathe in for the duration of one step and out for the duration of one step. In my life, I have been incredibly privileged to meet and train with several true, real deal masters. All of them had this one trait in common. They were patient; unafraid of boring their students. Unconcerned with appearances or entertainment, they delivered the material that would change lives, without apology or caveat.

Vladimir Vasiliev must have seen our faces on that first day. He must have known what we were thinking but somehow, he did not allow himself to be pulled into entertaining us at the expense of the training. I am deeply grateful.

BOX BREATHING

5-5-5-5

The count may consist of heartbeats, steps, or even seconds. It doesn't matter. An **even cadence** is what changes the physiology.

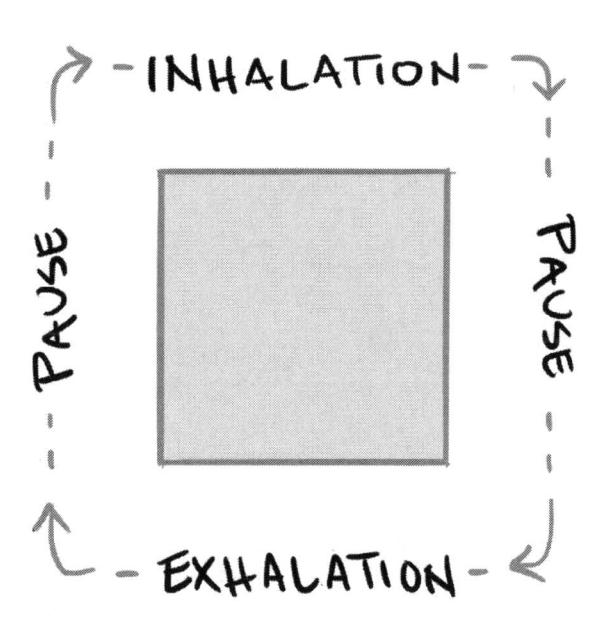

```
        → - INHALATION - ↘
      ↑                     ↓
      |                     |
    P |                     | P
    A |      [  square  ]   | A
    U |                     | U
    S |                     | S
    E |                     | E
      |                     |
      ↑                     ↓
        ← - EXHALATION - ↙
```

INHALE for 5 beats, **PAUSE** for 5 beats, **EXHALE** for 5 beats, **PAUSE** for 5 beats.

This is one example of box breathing or square breathing.

TRIANGLE BREATHING

The triangle pattern creates less internal pressure than square breathing. This breathing exercise is best after an injury to the torso.

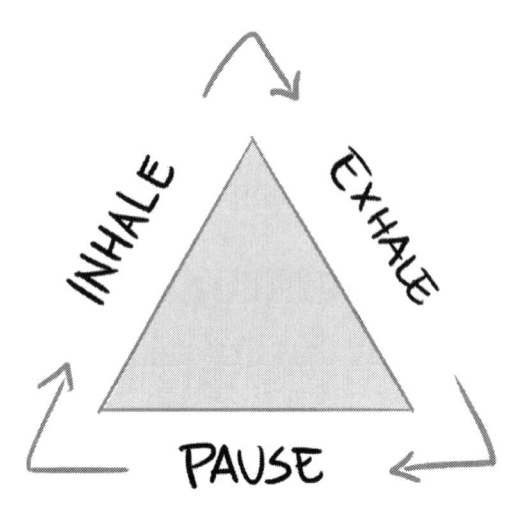

FAVORITE TRIANGLE BREATHING DRILL

INHALE for 3 heartbeats
EXHALE for 3 heartbeats

Pause and count heartbeats until you feel the first desire to breathe. This becomes the new number.

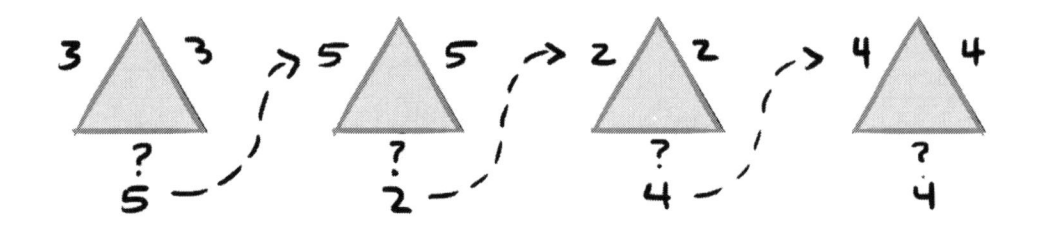

Walking and Breathing

To eliminate excess tension in the mind and body, walk and breathe.

A walking meditation

Drops of water hang from the bill of my cap. They look like diamonds in the streetlamp light, rubies if I encounter a red light and emeralds when the color says go. I love walking in the rain. The streets glitter, and the air is thick with mist. I know I shouldn't wear a hoodie, it blocks peripheral vision and dampens sound even more than the moisture heavy air, but I'm a big guy and I move pretty well so I figure I'm an unattractive target. Besides, it's too early for bad guys and I'm in an empty area and any other human presence would be as loud as a fog horn.

Striding down the deserted streets I focus my attention on moving gracefully. I have this idea that grace is defined as such because it means properly human. If you move the way we are designed to move, if you are connected to your body and can control its movement in multiple dimensions other humans perceive that as graceful. So, I move mindfully, as smoothly as I can, attempting with my whole demeanor, posture, speed and relaxed muscles to convey health, fluidity and power.

As I move through space I feel my guts moving gently up and down, pressing up on the diaphragm and then dropping down, leaving easy room for the diaphragm to move downwards. This gentle up and down movement of the diaphragm, driven by the movement of my viscera is in effect breathing me. It is a small breath, a small volume and if I am tense I cannot get enough air to sustain walking. But, if my timing is right and I am relaxed enough I can feel movement driving the breath. I begin to feel efficient, dangerous.

To explore more deeply I consider the heart muscle, pumping away in my chest, driving life giving oxygen and nutrients throughout my body. My heart lives in the same liquid, slippery cavity as my lungs and there is relationship between lungs, heart, diaphragm and legs. Stretching the crown of my head upwards into the low, rain pregnant sky, swinging my arms like pendulums, feeling how the movement first compresses then expands the thoracic cavity, timing the footfalls to the heart beat to the lung expansion to the pulsing that emanates from where I do not know, I find the bliss of movement and breath.

I don't remember any thought, only awareness and some feeling of gratitude and joy. To have a body, to breathe, to move, to be alive is a gift beyond my meager abilities to describe.

I don't know how long I walk this way. It is some timeless act to be breathed-moved, to measure it would be akin to asking the wind how far it has come, pointless.

Breath holding as a diagnostic

Somewhere I awaken as from a dream and stop. I've come a long way and it is time to turn towards home.

Inhale, exhale, pause...walking carefully, upright and relaxed, counting steps, the number does not matter it is only a relationship. In time the diaphragm muscle begins to convulse. The CO2 levels in my blood are telling the body that it must breathe. I am careful now, passing out and hitting my head on a curb would make for a tough evening. Still, I am waiting to inhale, waiting to feel that dark, tingling sensation that begins as a baseball sized round sensation; and then like black lightening or like a line of really fast ants, there is a clear movement from the point of origin of distress in a line to some exit point on my body. And then I inhale.

Continue walking, breathing in and out, listening and trying to find the recovery rhythm that is correct for this time, this night.

Inhale, exhale every step...every other step. Inhale for two steps, exhale for two steps.

Now inhale three steps, exhale three steps and switch to box breathing where the inhale, pause, exhale, pause pieces of the breath cycle are all the same.

Inhale 2 steps, exhale 3 steps...relaxing the body, dropping excess tension.

And then inhale 2 steps, exhale 2 steps getting the oxygen saturation levels up high so I can repeat the breath hold exercise twice more.

Three breath holds, three very long pauses after the exhale... each time noticing where the tension first arises. Moving the area of origin, breathing through the location where distress first began feels like a cleansing.

This is how you eliminate excess tension from the body and the mind.

Box breathing and walking

Box breathing, and walking is a standalone exercise. It is an extremely powerful exercise available to aid in the healing process. When I finish three cycles of breath hold, I move directly to box breathing.

Very simply, as diagrammed earlier, box breathing is considering four aspects of the breath cycle; an inhale, a pause, an exhale and another pause.

DRILL

To apply box breathing to walking you use your steps as the counting director.

For example: Inhale for 2 steps, pause for 2 steps, exhale for 2 steps, pause for 2 steps and then repeat. You are continuously walking, and your steps are creating the count mechanism.

I start with a 1 step box and work my way up to an uncomfortable count and then descend back down to the 1 step box.

You can consider each box as a rung on a ladder. I like to stay on each rung of the ladder for 7 repetitions of the same step count box.

Pulse Point Breathing

Here is a beautiful breathing exercise that will help you gain the body awareness necessary for breathing through obstruction to speed healing. This exercise was taught to me by Vladimir Vasiliev, a true master of breathwork and martial art.

Breathing, pulse points and pulse net:

When you are physically able, it is good to do tense and release exercises or walking or jogging to get the blood moving strongly before you begin this particular exercise. If you are unable to do any type of physical exertion you will need to be more patient and sensitive and aware of internal processes of your body. It is my experience that these are the most beautiful and productive times to train this breathing exercise.

DRILL

Lay down and get comfortable. Place the body in a neutral position with good alignment from head to toe and arms away from the body, palm up if possible. You can practice this exercise in any position or setting I am only suggesting an optimal scenario.

Close your eyes and begin breathing down into the lower abdomen to relax yourself.

Quiet your mind and bring it to focus on your heart muscle, the beating heart. Feel the size of your heart and its shape, feel it's rhythmic pulsing. Stay here with your heart for 10 or more beats.

Allow your attention to flow down from the heart muscle into the deep abdomen, towards the back. Find the aortic artery and feel it pulsing deep inside the upper abdomen. Stay there and feel the pulse for 10 or more beats.

Go lower with your awareness, locate the femoral arteries low in the pelvis, just before they reach out into the thighs, dual pulses. Stay connected to this pulse, aware of this pulse for 10 or more beats.

Allow your attention to rise up, visit the throat area and locate the carotid pulse in the arteries on either side. Pay attention to the new sensation, lighter, closer to the surface or whatever difference you may experience but stay focused on the pulse. Stay here for 10 or more beats.

Find the pulsing in your temple area, very light, very close to the surface. Stay with the pulsing for 10 or more beats.

Move to the brachial arteries, located on the inside of the upper arms. Feel the pulses here for 10 or more beats.

Follow the arteries out to the inside of the elbows and then the wrists and finally the hands. Locate and stay with the pulse in each of these areas for 10 or more beats.

Next, move your awareness back down, into the upper thighs and down to behind the knees. Locate and enjoy observing the pulse there in the popliteal area for 10 or more beats.

Follow the stream down inside the ankles and further to the feet themselves. Become aware of the pulsing sensation in both of your feet. Stay and absorb the experience of this pulsing for 10 or more beats.

And now comes the truly magical part of this exercise:

Expand your awareness to include all of the pulse points you have worked to discover and experience. All of the different points pulsing, are contained within the expanse of your awareness. You will find that the pulses are not simultaneous, but rather rocking...waving or pulsing through the body. We call this the pulse net. The connections between all the pulse points, the points themselves, illuminate your body in a different way. For me it is as if there is a golden web of moving and pulsing light encompassing and surrounding my body. The whole is larger than the individual pieces and I am aware of the space around my body as something that is beyond flesh or air. It is as if I witness the field of me, the golden light of me and healing is as natural as breathing.

PULSE POINTS

Pulse Points and the Pulse Net

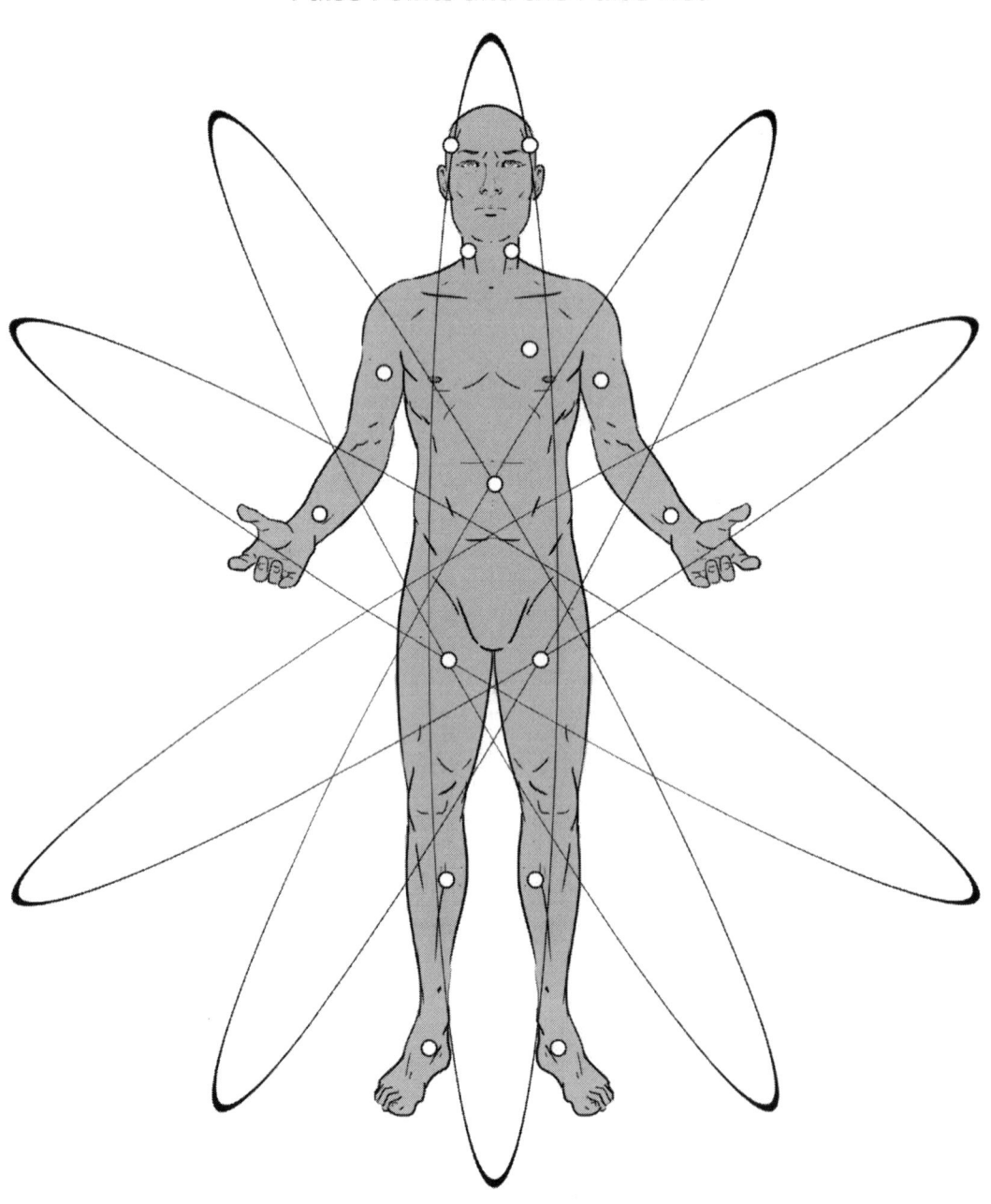

Free Breathing

or relaxed epiglottis breathing

DRILL

Relax your torso and throat, roll the shoulder and rotate the shoulder girdle relative to the pelvic girdle. When you perform this movement correctly, with relaxation and the correct rhythm you will be breathed by the movement of the torso. This is a fascinating experience. Air moves into and out of your lungs, one lung at a time, without the tensing and relaxing of the diaphragm muscle.

It feels as if the lungs are sponges and as one is squeezed and air moves out, the other is expanded and air moves into and fills the opening lung. As an experiment, I once punched a bag for fifteen minutes without intentionally activating my diaphragm muscle. That is to say, I moved vigorously for fifteen minutes without taking a breath. It was an intense exploration of breath sufficiency, continual breathing, relaxation and movement.

It is possible to bear crawl or jog and be breathed by the movement as well. Bear crawling is moving forwards, backwards or sideways with your hands and feet touching the ground, no knees please. Once you understand the concept and successfully practice it in one of these simpler movements you can begin to experiment and find movements that breathe you in many other contexts.

There are many benefits to this type of breathing, for example, you will be protected from sudden increases in intrathoracic pressure. If you are struck, if your torso's shape is suddenly changed by a twist or a tackle or some object smashing down on top of you, the air in your lungs will simply escape, reducing your risk of hernia or internal bleeding due to over pressured blood vessels.

But the practical benefits do not compare to the experience of realizing that breathing and moving are so profoundly connected that they may become indistinguishable. Imagine if you could move and breathe in ways that were synergistic instead of antagonistic to one another, your energy levels and your efficiency will increase dramatically. The experience of being breathed by your movement is almost magical.

As a practitioner of *taijiquan* I am often asked to show the proper breathing for the form and its many twisting movements. I always try to develop the idea that proper posture allows relaxation and with relaxation the movements themselves will breathe you. The principles and the movements embedded in the form will teach you to breathe correctly.

Conclusion

Inhaling we are born, exhaling our bodies pass into stillness. It is as if we exist for one breath and then disappear into the pause that follows.

Research continues into the benefits of various types or methods of breathing. Western scientists are only just beginning to understand how breathing impacts upon the vagus nerve, interacts with our hormonal systems, our blood chemistry and our abilities of the mind. It seems that the ancient yogis, qigong masters and martial artists were right all along, breathing really is the most important skill we can learn and practice.

This is a simple book of 30 breathing drills and a few stories to help illustrate the practice, for a more in-depth study of breathwork please consider reading my book "SHOT, Healing Hurt" or the book "Let Every Breath..." by Vladimir Vasiliev and Scott Meredith.

Made in the USA
San Bernardino, CA
05 November 2019